Cat First Aid: A Concise Qu

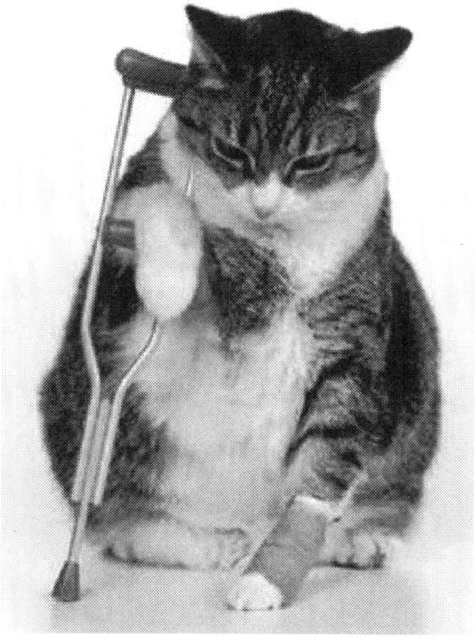

Table of Contents

FACTORS TO CONSIDER WHEN ADMINISTERING FIRST AID FOR YOUR CAT

What to do in a catastrophe

The average life expectancy of cats was about ten years just a few decades ago. Currently many live for close to 20 years through improved nutrition, vaccination and with improved standards of care. A large number of people keep their cats vaccinated by visiting veterinary services while maintaining regular treatment programs against parasites, for example, fleas, and worms.

However, a huge challenge is faced when deciding when a cat needs veterinary care for varying conditions and what conditions are termed as emergencies.

Before deciding if and when your cat needs veterinary care, it is important to undertake some few first aid measures.

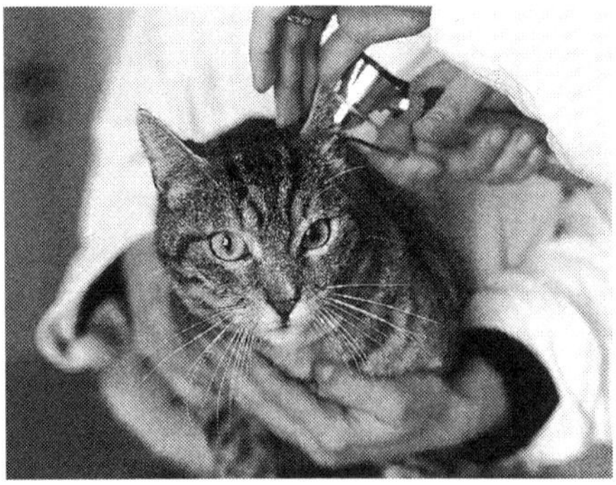

FIRST AID- THE BASICS

A lot of temptations are experienced when rushing into an emergency case without knowing what to do. Such is the case as it is human nature to try and help other living creatures who are in distress or agony. It, is, therefore essential to note that objectives of first aid are to preserve life and prevent further injury. In some situations, one may be able to provide first aid to the cat, while in others, especially if someone else is available to help, one should contact a veterinary officer immediately.

Rather than waiting for an incident to happen, it is important to learn when your cat is healthy and fit and also how to examine and restrain him. One should not try to do things all at once, though, and it is always good to reward your cat with play or food treats after an examination.

Restrain

As most cats hate being controlled it is fundamental that one uses minimum restraint. Wrap any injured or frightened cat with a towel or blanket when moving it. Subjecting a cat to restraints will cause him to bite, spit or hiss. If you are bitten or clawed, it is advisable that one seeks medical advice.

Also talk soothingly and approach the cat calmly, avoid eye contact so as not to threaten the cat and check the cat's expression.

Respiration

An average cat is capable of breathing 10 and 30 times a minute, while kittens have a faster respiratory rate than adult cats. A stressed cat, most, of the time, will have a higher respiratory rate than normal.

Once your cat is relaxed, watch its breathing in and out and count the number of times in 15 seconds. To find the rate per minute, multiply this by four. Such is not the case with fluffy cats as you may not be able to observe the chest movements. Placing a tissue paper in front of his nose will assist highly in counting the breaths, which is if the cat doesn't think that it's a game you were initiating.

It is not normal for a cat to breathe normally through its open mouth as this implies that extra effort is needed to breathe; hence this is wrong. Therefore, purring can cause challenge while trying to count the number of breathes a cat takes.

Heart Rate and Pulse

The resting heart rate of a healthy cat varies from 120 and 180 beats per minute, while kittens have a higher heart rate, which is up to 260 beats per minute. With your right hand, hold your cat under his chest and on the left side of his chest with your thumb and fingers on the right.

The heart rate tends to increase with excitement, exercise, fear, pain, shock, poisoning or attractive thyroid conditions, so it is fundamental that one determines the cat's heart rate when it is relaxed, fit and healthy.

Mucous Membrane Color and Capillary Refill Time

A healthy cat has moist and pink gums. A cat will have pale or white gums if it is losing blood or is in shock. A Yellow Tinge to its gums means that the cat is experiencing liver problems. Grey and blue gums show that the cat is receiving insufficient oxygen. In cases of heat stroke or carbon monoxide poisoning, a cat will have 'brick red" gums.

Observe your cat when he is healthy and see what shade of pink is normal for him.

ORDER OF IMPORTANCE

The emergencies listed in order of priority of action include the following: no pulse, no breathing, pulse but not breathing, unconscious, shock, breathing difficulties, chest puncture, severe bleeding, and abdominal puncture, extremely hot or extremely cold conditions, and poisoning.

Shock

White and rather pale gums, increased heart rate of more than 200 beats per minute and fast breathing of more than 40 beats per minute simply shock and must be dealt with whatever the emergency.

Bleeding, heart failure, burns, vomiting and diarrhea, trauma, diabetes, animal bites and many other causes are the causes of shock. It may lead to unconsciousness and death if left untreated. It is the first countermeasure in any emergency situation.

Early shock- is characterized by rapid breathing, high heart rate, pale or light colored mucous membranes and restlessness or lethargy.

Late shock- is characterized by an irregular heartbeat, shallow, and slow breathing, and lack of response, weakness or unconsciousness.

The following steps should be followed to minimize the effects of shock:

1. Place the cat on his side with his tail extended
2. Place a pillow behind his hind quarters
3. Apply pressure to stop bleeding
4. Prevent any heat loss by wrapping around a towel or an aluminum blanket
5. Contact the nearest vet immediately
6. Avoid giving food or water to the cat
7. If the cat is conscious, do not let it move around.

Anaphylactic shock- this can be caused by drugs, stings or insect bites or even food. In such cases, maintain an airway and give artificial respiration and heart massage if this two are required. By holding the hind limbs, suspend the cat for 10 seconds so as to prevent the lungs from filling with fluid. Allergic reactions to biting and injections cause the face to swell and itch; this condition can be rectified by giving the cat a steroid to reduce the effects of the foreign substance.

Artificial Respiration and Heart Massage

In cases where the heart or breathing has stopped, immediate provision of first aid may be life saving. This process of combining heart massage and artificial respiration is referred to as, cardiopulmonary resuscitation, which is commonly known as (CPR)

When dealing with a collapsed cat, look for the following signs of consciousness

1. If the cat responds when you clap your hands or whistle loudly
2. If the cat tries to bite you when you pinch hard between his toes
3. If the heart is beating but the cat is not breathing, a need for administration of artificial respiration is required.
4. Also if the heart is not beating and the cat is not breathing, CPR in such conditions is also required.

The process of Artificial respiration includes the following steps:

- To clear away any debris, put the cat on his side and move the neck forward
- Pull the cat's lips apart, place your mouth just over the cat's mouth.
- Blow in until the chest expands
- Take your mouth away and give the lungs time to deflate
- Repeat for every two to three seconds
- For every 10 seconds, check to ensure that the heart is still beating
- Seek veterinary care

The process of chest massage includes the following:

- To try and direct more blood to the brain, place the cat on its side with the head lower than the body.
- Hold the cat's chest between your thumbs as your fingers hold the elbows
- So as to compress the chest, squeeze upwards towards the neck.
- Repeat the pumping action about 100 times a minute.
- Get veterinary attention immediately

Wounds

1. Bruises

Often caused by trauma to the skin without breaking the skins surface, they can be severe or superficial. It may be hard to see the effects of a bruise especially in darkly pigmented cats. Bruises bring about swelling, pain and skin discoloration.

To help reduce swelling, apply a cold compress such as an ice pack to the affected area so as to avoid damage from the cold. In situations of bruising to the abdomen, consult a veterinary officer immediately.

2. Cuts

Here the skin is broken, and the tissues exposed to dirt and bacteria which is a high risk of infection. With a non-stick absorbent material apply direct pressure to stop the bleeding and in cases of severe bleeding do not remove the blood soaked absorbing material so as to avoid further bleeding. Wrap the wound with a bandage and seek veterinary services immediately.

However, if there is a lot of hair adjacent to the wound, one should either cut it with scissors before dressing the wound or apply it with KY jelly to the actual wound once you're through with cleaning and clip the hair.

To avoid damaging the sensitive tissue, do not use antiseptic solutions to clean wounds. Apply Pressure with a bandage and immediate veterinary attention is sought to wounds that continue to bleed even after administration of pressure.

3. Abscesses

Abscesses are mostly observed in cats that tend to fight; these cats regularly suffer from ulcers which are brought about by teeth punctures introducing bacteria under the skin. Pain and discharge of purse is observed around the affected area.

It's essential to seek veterinary services as a course of antibiotics needs to be prescribed to the cat. In most cases, abscesses will swell but not discharge and in such situations, a cat may need sedating, and the abscesses drained.

Bandaging

Cats do not like to feel as if they are being restrained, and hence, any bandaging will be difficult to administer in any fully conscious cat. It is important to bandage your cat as this keeps the wound dry and protected from further injury. If your cat uses a litter tray, cover the bandage with a plastic bag to avoid it getting wet, keep your cat indoors and monitor it regularly.

It is also advisable not to apply a splint to a conscious cat as it is expected to struggle too much and cause further damage to the wound. Place a small T-shirt over the cats head and wrap the whole trunk and affected limb in the T-shirt and remove the affected limb in situations where for example, an arm is dangling.

Transporting an Injured Cat

To protect yourself and the cat from any injuries, care must be taken when lifting and transporting an injured cat. Injured cats tend to scratch and bite especially if it's still in shock

Minor Injuries

If the cat can get into the box or container, it is advisable to offer support as you let him do so. Lift the cat gently by placing one arm under his chest and at the same time use your other hand to cradle the body.

Critical Injuries

These are injuries where a cat is unable to move for himself for example fractures and paralysis. Keep any legs uppermost as you support the back. In cases of chest injuries, the damaged lung should be on the side the cat is laying. Cover the box to prevent heat loss as you place the cat in its transport. Make sure there is no pressure on his chest and that he can breathe freely in case of any wrapping.

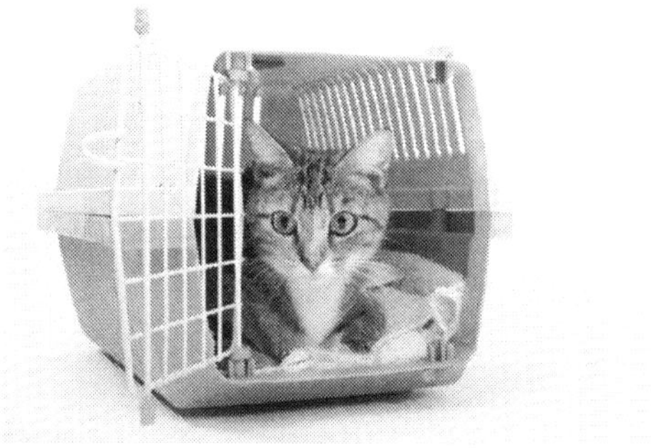

SITUATIONS THAT REQUIRE VETERINARY SERVICES AND ATTENTION

If your cat is experiencing severe pain or injuries that put its life in danger, then it's important to seek medical care.

1. Body Temperature

The standard body temperature of a cat is around 38.1 and 39.2 degrees Celsius, that is 100.5 to 102.5 degrees Fahrenheit.

Nervousness, exercise, excess heat, and infection can cause temperatures to be above normal, while exposure to cold weather and shock can cause temperatures to be below normal. One should never take cats temperatures by mouth. Use the rectal area instead by lubricating the tip of a glass thermometer with KY jelly and insert it about 2cm into the cat's rectum. Wait for of 60-90 seconds, remove and read the findings.

Temperatures above 40.6 to 41 degrees Celsius indicate high temperatures and immediate veterinary services should be sought after. Probable cases of fever can be observed by temperatures above 39.4 degrees Celsius and in this case, veterinary services need to be seeked the same day.

Temperatures below 37.8 degrees Celsius also require seeking of veterinary services.

2. Behavior

A change to your cat's normal behavior is a cause for concern. Also, unexpected purring can show pain or distress, and it is essential not to assume that a purring cat is happy.

If a cat does not respond to your interaction, it may be due to drowsiness, depression, and instability. It is, therefore, important to check the color of the cat's gums, pulse, and breathing rate. White gums mean your cat is in shock and needs veterinary care immediately.

When a cat responds with resentment, vocalization or tries to hide once you touch him, then this means that he may have an injury or be going through pain. It is, therefore, advisable to seek veterinary attention the same day.

In situations such as labored breathing, sucking chest sounds or gagging, exaggerated swallowing, decreased alertness, decreased sleeping and restlessness and coughing it is essential to seek medical and veterinary services.

3. Breathing

In cases such as gasping, labored, shallow, rapid or very slow breathing, wheezing, coughing, intense panting, distressed, pawing at the mouth, gagging, profuse saliva and choking, one should administer first aid and seek veterinary services in less than 12 hours.

Too much pressure can cause internal bleeding and hence, it is essential to give CPR and seek veterinary attention immediately.

4. Mobility and General Appearance

Look for any presence of blood and any visible wound. Broken teeth and nails can show possible road traffic accidents and also the potential for more severe injuries. It is, therefore, important to check for signs of shock such as pale gums, high respiratory and pulse rate, in which case immediate veterinary attention need to be sort after.

The following conditions require veterinary services: muscle spasm, slow, deliberate movement, dilated pupils, swelling, threads or strings from mouth to anus, arched back, tilted head and circling.

5. Odors

It is advisable to seek veterinary services if your cat has a smell to his breath. Also, if you can smell antifreeze or tar on your cat as well as smoke, if you smell urine, or if feces or blood are present on the coat then in this situation check for injuries and treat as necessary.

6. Dehydration

To assess levels of dehydration check for “skin tenting,’ you should pinch the skin between the cat’s shoulder blades wherein normal animals the skin will spring back into position but in dehydrated animals, the skin will remain tented. Where the eyeballs recede into the cat’s head, check that the eyes do not appear sunken as this is an indicator of marked dehydration.

Potential causes of dehydration include not drinking/eating, vomiting, diarrhea, excessive panting and loss of body fluids.

Seek immediate veterinary attention for marked dehydration, and it is likely that a drip of intravenous fluid is to be administered to your cat. With ill or very young animals, it can be quite challenging and hence, sometimes the fluids are given under the skin.

7. Eye Conditions

It is important that one looks for discharge, cloudiness, bleeding or injury as the eye is very prone to such injuries. Dilated pupils mean fear, pain, excitement, sudden blindness or shock in brightly lit areas. Therefore, make a movement towards each of your cat's eye with a finger and if your cat can see the finger, it will blink.

For signs such as the eye hanging out, bleeding, swelling or severe bruising around the eye, the pupils are dilated, and evidence of shock are present and if your cat appears to be suddenly blind, seek immediate veterinary care.

Cloudy eyes and failure for the cat to open his eyes need veterinary attention within less than 12 hours. Likewise, unequal pupil sizes, discharge of green or yellow substances from the eyes, if the third eyelid is visible, if your cat is constantly rubbing his eyes all require veterinary care within less than 24 hours.

8. Ear conditions

Signs of concussion are possible are likely to be observed in case of bleeding from either ears or nose after trauma, in which case immediate veterinary services are required. It is essential to examine the ear canals for swelling, discharge or pain and if your cat is moving his head up and down and left and right, followed by a waxy or smelly discharge, seek veterinary services immediately.

EXAMINATION OF BODY PARTS

Examination of The Head and Neck

In most cases, there will be limited evidence of injuries caused by concussions, and hence, one should examine the head, jaws, and cheeks for swelling or heat. To see if the cat is in pain, move the head from side to side and up and down. Also, feel the area around the neck for stickiness that may show a puncture wound.

Examination of The Chest, Abdomen and Legs

To feel for heat sensitivity or body fluids run your hands over the cat's back, chest and groin. In cases of cat bites, the surrounding area will be sticky and will also discharge fluid. Look for bruising by parting the hair as you examine each leg in turn noticing any damage to the nails. Note any evidence of pain or heat as you bend and flex each joint.

Urinary problems can be life threatening if the bladder becomes distended with urine during blockage and hence, it is important to check and feel your cat's bladder when he is relaxed.

Examination of Tail, Anus and Genitals

A common site for bite wounds is mostly at the base of the tail. It is, therefore, important that one is thorough when doing a check-up around this area. Observe also if the cat lashes out, and there shouldn't also be areas of heat or prominent bumps.

If a limp tail doesn't respond, there might be a likelihood of a spinal cord injury.

The anus should always be clean, and any pungent smell along the anal glands mean that your cat may have possible injuries, so it is advisable to look for further signs of damage or shock.

Lastly, examine the vagina and penis for evidence of inflammation or discharge.

The Skin and Fur

A well-kept cat with smooth and sleek fur may suddenly become unkempt and untidy; in this case, the cat should be checked for possible signs of injury or illness.

Seek immediate medical attention to a cat that might have all of a sudden started scratching or biting and showing signs of mutilation.

Check for fleas on cats within 24 hours and application of an anti-parasiticide is approved if the condition persists.

See a veterinary officer if the swellings or lumps appear suddenly within 24 hours and if the lumps and swellings take time before they form, see a veterinary officer soon.

Grease residue or oil on your cat are signs of injury, and one should check if the cat is breathing normally.

The Alimentary System

Some gastrointestinal problems can be quite serious. Seek prompt medical advice if the cat is vomiting or passes diarrhea that is bloody or black, especially if the vomiting is persistent and diarrhea explosive.

If your cat has vomited and had diarrhea which continues after 24 hours and loss of appetite for 24 hours, then one should seek immediate veterinary care.

If your cat has lost weight, drinking more or less than usual or a change in excretion is noticed, then immediate veterinary services are required.

The Bladder

If a cat is straining but unable to urinate or hasn't passed urine within 24 hours, then in this case immediate veterinary services are required. Likewise, seek a veterinary officer if your cat is urinating more frequently than usual, is urinating in inappropriate areas, has blood present in urine or seems incontinent.

COPING IN EMERGENCY SITUATIONS

It is essential first to assess the cat's condition and situation when an emergency arises. However, one should take care as not to endanger himself or the cat. Therefore seek immediate veterinary attention if the cat is in pain, collapsed, is in distress, showing signs of shock, the cat is unable to move, visible injuries, cases of poisoning, head trauma, and breathing difficulties.

Problems with Kittening

Sometimes the owner of the cat may not realize that the cat was pregnant until the day they are born, as most cats can kitten without any assistance.

However, complications arise if: no labor is apparent after 66 days of pregnancy, the cat fails to produce a kitten within one hr of the first water bag being seen, and the cat fails to go into labor within 24 hours,

Likewise, failure to deliver a kitten after 45 minutes of steady contractions, more than 2hrs passing before the last kitten was born, cases of bleeding during pregnancy, smelly discharge is passed during labor. In these situations, immediate veterinary services should be sought.

In cases where a kitten has gotten stuck in the birth canal, gently hold it with a clean, warm towel, apply steady traction on and arc towards the mother's hind feet until delivery of the kitten. Also, seek veterinary attention if there is resistance or if the kitten is presented with the hind legs first.

In situations where mothers do not show interest with the newborn kitten, the following measures should be undertaken: rub the kitten's body to stimulate breathing, wipe around the kittens face removing fluid from the nostrils and use a clean towel to remove the membranes from the kitten's nose and head.

When breathing is not forthcoming, hold the kitten firmly between your cupped hands and from the shoulder height down in an arc, swing rapidly to expel fluid from the air passages. Stop when the kitten moves or cries.

The mother should lick the kittens and encourage them to suckle immediately after birth. Consult a veterinary officer if the mother is staggering or trembling, straining to urinate, has lack of appetite, is producing a foul-smelling vaginal discharge or has hard painful mammary glands

Burns

1st Degree burns where the skin is intact and damaged by heat, in such situations, flush the affected area with clean water as soon as possible, cover with a non-stick bandage to protect the area and to prevent the cat from biting. Change the dressing daily and seek a veterinary officer in extreme conditions.

Where the skin is intact but burned by chemicals, flush the area for close to 20 minutes if your cat will tolerate this. Using one teaspoon baking soda per pint of water flush the foreign substance, especially if it is a known chemical and cover with a non-stick dressing.

2nd Degree (partial) 3rd Degree (total) Burns, such are cases where the skin barrier is breached

Constipation

Constipation is usually due to hairs and feces that are too dry to pass through the anus. Other causes of constipation also include hernias, tumors and ingested bones and grass. Constipation is most common in older cars and preparations of liquid paraffin can help keep the stools softened.

Seek a veterinary service, if in 24hrs the cat is in pain, vomiting, passing out ribbon-like foul smelling feces. If the feces are stuck in the hair around the anus, trim carefully with scissors and wash the area and also if the grass is protruding from the cat's anus, gently ease it out.

Convulsions/Seizures

Convulsions are usually conditions that can cause cats to start fitting and cats which experience this regularly are called epileptic. Other causes include low glucose in the blood, low blood calcium, and liver complications.

The general signs and symptoms of seizures is a collapsed cat or a twitching cat which is often lying by its side.

It is important not to panic once a cat seems to be having a convulsion and it is very rare for a cat to choke on its tongue, hence, avoid putting your fingers near the cat's mouth as you may get bitten.

Try also to distract your cat if you see that he is having a mild convulsion as this will prevent a full seizure.

Also, reduce light levels and background noise. If the seizures stop within four minutes, reassure the cat and keep him in a quiet area where you can monitor him.

Seek immediate veterinary service if the seizure continues for longer than four minutes or seems to stop then start again.

Coughing

Unwanted materials from the air passages are removed through coughing. Instances of a cat coughing can be caused by allergies, infection, pollen, chest disease tumors or fluids in the lungs. See veterinary services immediately if a cough is causing breathing difficulties or there is a blood tinged material coughed up.

Consult a veterinary officer within 24 hours in cases where your cat is experiencing high temperatures, weight loss, lethargy, loss of appetite and following exposure to smoke.

Fill the room with steam if the cat is experiencing a dry and unproductive cough. If the cough does not improve for three days, seek veterinary services.

Diabetes Emergencies

Cases of diabetes emergencies when either too much or too little of insulin has been administered to the cat; if untreated it can lead to death.

A cat is likely to be hypoglycemic if its starts twitching and convulsing, becomes weak and changes its normal behavior. It is, therefore, important to keep glucose or honey on hand if these signs are evident. Give liquid glucose into the cat's mouth immediately. If the seizures continues, rub glucose syrup on the gums and seek immediate veterinary assistance and always make sure that your cat has eaten a meal before administering insulin.

Your cat may be diabetic if it is eating and drinking more than usual but still losing weight, and hence, seek a veterinary officer immediately.

Smell the breath of your cat if it is vomiting or has a sweet fruity smell as it is likely to be hypoglycemic and if so, seek immediate veterinary care.

Diarrhea

Diarrhea is a common condition which is caused by diet changes or allergies. It can also be caused by infections, metabolic problems or tumors.

Seek immediate veterinary services if the following conditions are observed: diarrhea that is bloody, explosive, accompanied by vomit, causing dehydration and is making the cat weak or depressed.

If your cat is otherwise healthy, provide plenty of drinking water and remove food for 12 hours, Give kaolin mixture such as Kaogel, if diarrhea persists for more than 24 hours or blood is present, seek immediate veterinary services.

Give your cat a small amount of cooked white fish or chicken after 12 hours of fasting. Continue with small amounts of cooked white fish or chicken.

Once you change your cat's diet, it's important to do it gradually so as not to upset the gut bacteria and cause diarrhea.

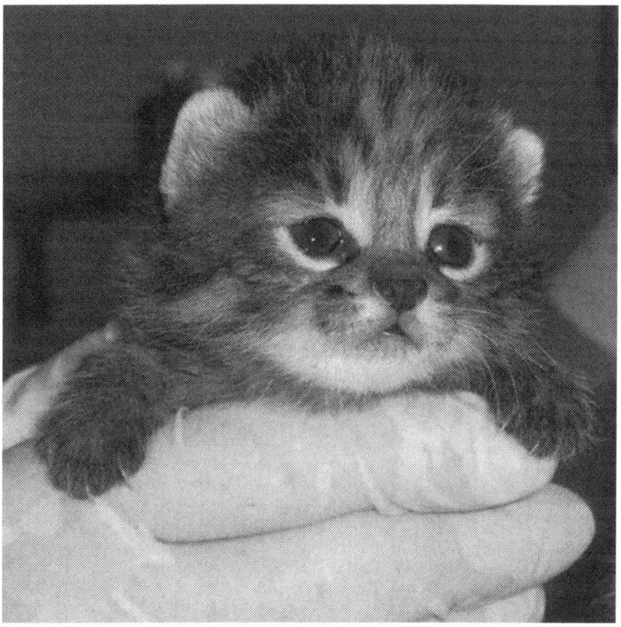

Drowning

Drowning is rare as most cats tend to avoid water but can happen if a cat falls into deep water. In such situations, one should rescue the cat, if the cat is conscious, keep it warm and wrap it in a towel and if the cat is unconscious, hold it upside down and swing it from side to side, gently, so as to drain the lungs of the water.

Also, position the cat on his side with his head lower than the chest, clear any debris from the mouth and remove the tongue forward and begin CPR if there is no heartbeat.

In occurrences where the cat is not breathing, give artificial respiration. Lastly, it is also essential to seek veterinary attention and care.

Electric Shock

Electric shocks are mostly caused when a cat chews through an electric cable. Any electric shock can trigger cardiac arrest and burns to the affected part of the body. Avoid putting yourself in danger by ensuring that the power source in your house is turned off. To move the cat away from the incidence of shock, use a wooden broom and apply cold compresses to burns to minimize further damage. It is also fundamental to watch for signs of shock developing.

Keep kittens away from electric cords to prevent incidents, and apply butter spray to the cords as a deterrent and reposition or box in cords that look tempting to play with.

Ear Injuries

Bandage the year as ear as you can if the flap is bleeding; avoid using too much dressing as it can prevent the cat from breathing properly.

Cases where the cat is shaking his head, scratching at the ear or holding the ear lower on one side he may have a foreign body in the ear, ear mites or may suffer from infection, symptoms such as loss of balance and co-ordination may mean that your cat is suffering from an inner ear problem, and hence, the cat should be taken to a veterinary services as soon as possible.

Eye Injuries

Eye injuries are very critical if left untreated. A small scratch on the eye may cause a lot of complications including loss of vision or sight if left untreated. Therefore, immediate veterinary attention must be sought in case of the following symptoms and conditions:

A. Eyeballs out of their socket- in this case, do not try to push back in but instead, cover with a clean, soft damp cloth, ideally soaked in warm saline. Get to the veterinary as soon as possible as every second counts in eye injuries.
B. Damage on the surface of the eye
C. Blood in the eye or a foreign body-to avoid further injury if you cat is rubbing at the eye, apply an Elizabeth collar.

D. Irregular pupils- check for signs of trauma and other injuries.
E. If the eye is closed and painful
F. If one eye looks longer than the other.

Chemical burns- use saline if available or water to irrigate the eye for at least 5 minutes. To prevent your cat from rubbing his eyes on the way to the veterinary, use an Elizabeth collar. Take long along any packaging related to the chemical.

Veterinary services should be sought within 24 hours if there is a green and yellow discharge from an eye or the eyes seem inflamed and bloodshot. Clear the discharge gently by bathing with cooled-down boiled water. If the discharge is clear or colorless, or if your cat is sneezing and rubbing his face, these may be signs of an allergic reaction, and in such situations seek instant veterinary attention.

Fainting

Fainting rarely occurs in cats but it is more likely to occur in flat-faced breeds such as Persians. Fainting is normally caused by a temporary deficit of oxygen or sugar. Causes of fainting can be due to low blood glucose or coughing as well as a heart disease.

A cat will first start by being weak and uncoordinated, collapse into unconsciousness and recover within minutes.

However, it is important to ensure that the tongue is removed outwards to create a clear airway and check for any signs of shock. Keep your cat quiet for one hour following the faint. Lastly, seek veterinary care if the condition persists or in such recurrent episodes.

Fish hooks can become embedded in the paws, lips, tongue, stomach if swallowed and it is very fundamental to note that one should never remove the fish hook stuck in the cats' mouth as this may lead to further damage or injury. In case you suspect that your cat has swallowed a fish hook, seek a veterinary surgeon immediately.

If the hook is on an external part such as the rib or paw, the barb of the fishing hook should be cut off with wire cutters and the hook removed out in the direction to which it entered.

Fractures

It is essential to seek medical services in cases of fracture; the cat may experience the following problems;

A. An arched back, is in extreme pain or is paralyzed. Transport the cat on a flat board.
B. The cat probably has a broken bone if a cracking sound was heard at the time of injury, a broken bone is visible, a limb is hanging, and there is sudden swelling.
C. Hard bulges on the chest walls are as a result to rib injuries and fractures. Torn sheets are hence wrapped around a cat's chest, starting with the area of the soft

bulge. The dressing should not interrupt with the breathing.

Frostbite and Hypothermia

Hypothermia can result when a body is exposed to chill or extremely cold conditions. Ears and tail are more prone to suffer from hypothermia since they have little protection.

Cases of frostbite are characterized by pale or red and puffy extremities as well as pain when these extremities are touched. If the core temperature drops significantly, life is threatened. Immersion in cold water also causes hypothermia.

Seek immediate veterinary attention in case of shock, keep the cat warm during transport, and wrap the cat loosely in bubble wrap with a tin foil then with a thin blanket and keep the ambient temperature warm.

Your vet may need to provide warm fluids and drinks which will continue the process of slowly re–heating the cat.

If extensive damage is sustained for a prolonged period, the skin may die, and the area may need to be surgically removed, in order for the frostbite to recover and to improve blood flow.

Heart Failure

Most cats do not experience cases of heart failure as most cats can compensate up to a certain point even with a failing heart. However, the initial signs may present very suddenly when the cat is unable to cope, and one of the most common symptoms is breathing difficulties due to the accumulation of fluid in the lungs of the cat.

Immediate veterinary services should be sought if the cat is scratching or biting as well as showing signs of distress with his breathing. If the cat has collapsed and is not breathing, it is important to give CPR and immediately seek veterinary help.

Heatstroke

In such conditions, cats generally have inadequate means of losing body heat through panting and sweating through their pads. If the surrounding temperature is too high, body temperature rises rapidly, and death quickly follows. The warm interior of tumble dryers is attractive to cats, therefore, ensure that your cat us not inside before closing the door and switching on the drier.

Signs of heat stroke include panting and a glazed expression, copious salivation, red gums, increased heart rate, rectal temperature of 40.6 degrees Celsius.

In such conditions, the cat should be removed from the hot environment immediately, it's body (but not its head) immersed in cool freezing water and also encouraged to drink small amounts of cold water.

Other methods of countering heat stroke include taking regular temperature checkups until it has fallen to below 39.4 degrees Celsius, treat shock and seek immediate medical attention for your cat, massage the legs gently vigorously to aid in circulation as well as reducing the risks of shock and it is important for your vet to administer cold drinks and fluids to further lower the temperature.

A major point to note is that one should never give Aspirin to a cat in order to reduce the cat's temperature.

Injury to Skin

If symptoms of shock are present, seek immediate veterinary services, and one shouldn't make inaccurate assumptions. Look for any signs of bruising, abrasion or puncture if your cat avoids any contact with you such as touching. In situations where there is a small cut, remove the hair adjacent to the cut slowly and carefully and clean the wound with salt water.

Cases of injury to skin that may require medical attention include the following: wounds caused by a knife or sharp objects, ongoing bleeding after three minutes of applied pressure, signs of shock, abnormal breathing, obvious pains and distress and bites by other animals.

It is essential to note that one should never remove a penetrating object as this may cause injury to arteries and veins causing further bleeding, instead, move the cat with the object in it.

In cases of impalement on railings get a veterinary surgeon to assist you in the matter. Death can result when an inserted object is removed from a cat and such situations are very fatal.

It is vital to perform thorough examinations if you suspect your cat to be suffering from severe grave injuries and traumatic experiences. Lastly, seek medical and veterinary attention for your cat.

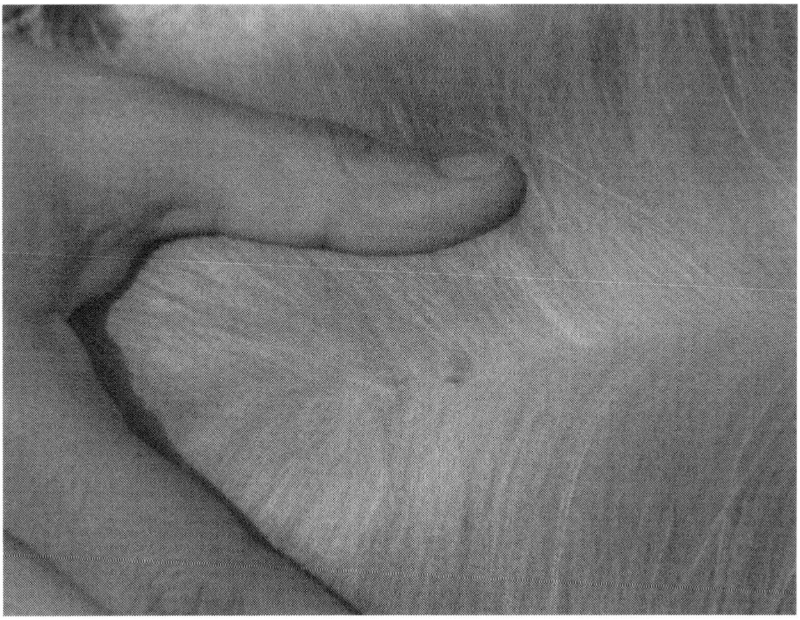

Lameness

Lameness is caused by fractures, dislocations, sprains and strains. Instant veterinary attention should be sought after in such situations. Pain, distress, and sudden weakness, visible bones, and abdominal bends to the limp are likely to cause lameness and require immediate care from medical practitioners.

Within 24 hours if a joint is hot, painful swollen, or the cat is unable to bear weight, these are signs of a possible injury and veterinary care is required to cure this problem. Likewise, if your cat is in shock, seek medical attention for your cat.

Drugs such as Paracetamol are not suitable for cats and hence, administering them will can lead to death or cause further injuries.

Rest your cat and observe him for close to 48 hours if he continues to show normal behavior but has developed a sudden limp. Also keep your cat indoors in lameness conditions as releasing him outdoor will hinder his ability from escaping from danger which further leads to further injuries.

As in the case of older cats, many have arthritic changes going on their hind limbs and spines, and your vet can prescribe routine drugs which can help with the relief pain and inflammation.

Losing Balance

Methods which may cause a cat to lose its balance include the following: concussions, diabetic crisis, shock and ear infections as well as vestibular diseases (conditions of the inner year).

Symptoms such as increased thirst and weight loss are likely to be signs of diabetes while shaking and scratching of the head are signs of possible ear injuries.

Veterinary services should be sought after in cases the eyes are moving from side to side either quickly or slowly. Ensure that your cat doesn't injure or cause further damages to himself if he seems out of balance. Lastly, all cases of loss of balance should be taken seriously, and veterinary services should be visited immediately.

Mouth Conditions

Cats do not normally drop their food while eating or drool saliva as well as showing signs of pain when his jaws are opened or when his mouth is touched. Likewise, bad breath is highly unlikely in cats and can be because of a tooth root infection, gingivitis, presence of a foreign body or a tumor. If bleeding is present, check to see whether your cat is exhibiting signs of shock or any other injuries.

Kittens often bleed from their mouth during teething periods. Also if your cat is showing signs of increased hunger but is unable to eat, seek medical attention as this may be due to a possible injury or swelling in the mouth region.

Nasal Problems

Cats are prone to nose injuries as they most of the times get foreign objects in them. They might show signs of possible nasal injuries such as presence of a foreign object by squeezing, possibly pawing at the face, difficulty swallowing and a discharge from the nostrils, with possible blood stains.

Your veterinary surgeon is most likely going to apply an anesthesia to your cat so as to look up the nose and back of the throat and may also need to take some radiographs. Once the foreign objects are removed, cats tend to recover properly.

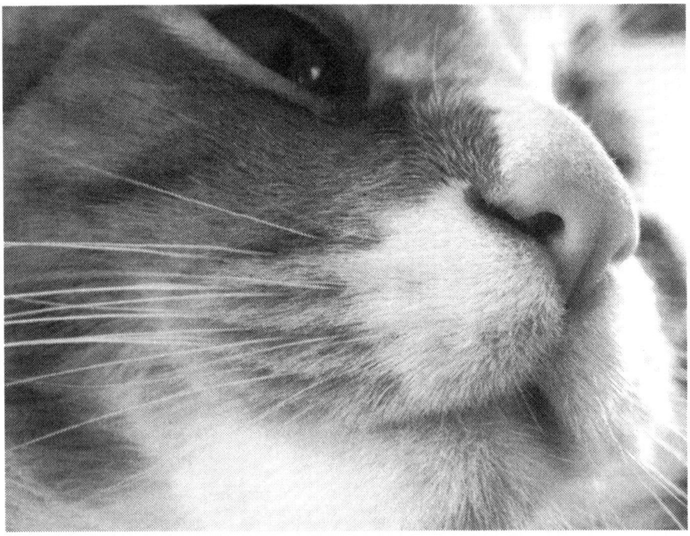

Skin Contact

An example of causes of skin poisoning is mostly through chemicals which the cats rub against their skin. Systemic poisoning also occurs because, the cat may try to reduce the burning effects of the chemicals by licking and hence, causing further poisoning and infection to the mouth region. If cases of shock, convulsions, and pain become apparent, seek immediate medical attention for your cat.

One can remove the contamination if the cat has not shown signs of distress or pain and has not licked the affected area. Wear gloves and apply a significant amount of vegetable oil in situations where a cat has gone into contact with paint, tar or motor oil. Cut the hairs if the skin condition has hardened instead of softening and removing.

Flush the area with water for about 5-15 minutes if the contamination has been caused by anything other than paint, tar or petroleum.

It is very essential to note that, one should not use paint stripper, turpentine, methylated spirit or concentrated biological detergent to remove the contamination. Likewise, never use flea treatments indicated for dogs or cats as it contains Permethrin which is toxic and causes death to cats.

Inhaled

Inhaled poisons interfere with the overall breathing of the cat, trigger shock, inflame the respiratory tract and can also affect the eyes. Symptoms include unconsciousness, un-coordination, deep red gums, breathing difficulties and coughing with or without expulsion of blood.

Inhaled poisons may include smoke and carbon monoxide caused by house fires and car engine batteries respectively.

It is, therefore, advisable that for inhaled toxins and fumes, ensure appropriate aeriation so as to improve the air circulation and improve the breathing rate of your cat.

Swallowed

Cats are very cautious about what they eat but can swallow poisons if medicines prescribed for other animals or human beings are fed to them knowingly or unknowingly. Also as mentioned earlier, through also licking chemicals from their skins so as to decrease the effects of chemical burns, can cause poisoning.

Immediate veterinary attention is required if your cat exhibits signs such as unconsciousness, has stopped breathing, is experiencing seizures and convulsions, may have taken in an alkaline or acidic substance and most importantly if your cat is in shock.

Discourage vomiting in instances where the following substances may have been injested: caustic soda, chlorine bleach, dishwasher granules, drain cleaner, kerosene or paraffin, laundry detergents, lye, oven cleaners, paint stripper and remover, paint thinner, petrol, furniture, floor or shoe polish, toilet cleaner, and wood preservative.

Acid poisons

Here, one is required to administer the following: egg white, bicarbonate of soda, charcoal powder or olive oil by mouth.

Alkaline poisons

For alkaline poisons, give egg white, vinegar or citrus fruit juice in small amounts. Also, pour vinegar on alkali burns to the skin and the mouth and lastly, seek medical services and veterinary care.

A major point to also note is that if your cat has ingested a substance other than an acid, alkali or petroleum based within the last two hours, seek immediate medical advice and care.

Precautions to take include draining cleaner, solvents, paint stripper products with acid or alkali symbols on the label. Such chemical substances are prone to poison the cats in particular through licking contaminated areas of their fur. Lastly, is to get immediate veterinary help.

Poisoning also occurs if the cats lick the insecticides from their coats and further and end up poisoning themselves.

Ingested carbonates cause: agitation, restlessness, twitching, salivation, convulsions and comas, while organ phosphates cause, hind leg weakness, breathing difficulties, muscle tremors, salivation and increased urination and defection.

Rodent Poison

When visiting a veterinary officer because of this problem, it is important to look for the name of the poison or bring a sample of the container to the veterinary officer. A major fact to note is that cats are also poisoned by eating prey which has been contaminated with a rodenticide.

Common rat poisons such as Warfarin can cause vomiting, lethargy, signs of internal bleeding, pale gums, and signs of shock a well as bruises on skins. Once you discover that a cat has swallowed a rodent poison, induce vomiting then administer activated charcoal into the mouth. Lastly, is to seek immediate medical attention.

Poisons such as strychline can cause: tenseness or stiffness, convulsions and one should visit veterinary attention as strychline can be very fatal.

Also, sodium fluoroacetate can cause: initial excitement followed by depression, seizures, vomiting, increased urination and defecation. In such cases, it is important to induce vomiting and give activated charcoal.

Slug and Snail Bait-Metaldehyde

Cats are unlikely to eat Metaldehyde on their own accord but may eat slugs infected by the poison. Metaldehyde causes Tremors, salivation, convulsions, and comas.

If recently swallowed, that is within 2 hours, induce vomiting and seek immediate veterinary attention.

Antifreeze-Ethylene Glycol

It is a generally fatal condition and can cause death if not action upon in good time. The cat tends to lick car radiators as they are very appealing. Symptoms include the following: wobbling, convulsions, vomiting, collapsing, acute renal failure, comas, and death.

It is important to induce vomiting and administer activated charcoal. Also seek immediate veterinary attention and if you're a long distance away from veterinary services, administer a small amount of alcohol by mouth.

Aspirin

As mentioned earlier, the most common cause of poisoning is when owners give human medications and prescriptions to cats, thinking that they are helping in relieving the pain.

Aspirin may cause loss of appetite, depression, abdominal cramp, vomiting with or without stains of blood and un-coordination of movements.

If the cat ingests aspirin accidentally, it is advisable first to induce vomiting with washing crystals (e.g. Lectric), give no further medication immediately seek medical care for your cat.

Illegal Drugs, For Example, Cannabis and Ecstasy
Cats also get poisoned once they take in cannabis or any other illicit drug and show signs of this by becoming uncoordinated, agitated, fear biting and dilated pupils.

It is very essential to seek medical attention and avoid unnecessary sensory stimulation with light and sound.

Sedatives, Antidepressants and Anti Anxiety Drugs
If left around, prescription medications can be ingested by cats, or when administered to the cat intentionally, they cause staggering, depression, restlessness, erratic heartbeat, deep sleep or coma.

Keep your cat warm and consult your veterinary officer immediately for advice.

IMPORTANT POINTS TO REMEMBER

- Do not give prescription medications to your cat

- Garden and garage chemicals, as well as cleaning products, should be kept out from the reach of cats.
- Keep your cat out of the area when using weed killer or pest poison and also remember to follow the required instructions
- Insecticidal products indicated for other animals should not be used on cats
- All animal and human medication should be carefully labeled and kept in their original containers and away from the reach of children. **Poisonous plants**

Cats are known to play, chew and eat plants in the house and the garden area. Some very dangerous plants include Castrol oil plant, dumb cane, mistletoe, thorn apple or jimsonweed, cherry laurel, hemlock, ivy leaves and berries, lilies, oleander, and yew.

Others also include amaryllis, autumn, crocus, bleeding heart, bloodroot, flower bulbs of any kind, foxglove, Jerusalem, larkspur, lily of the valley, mushrooms, rhubarb, stinging nettle, Virginia creeper, azalea, box, chinaberry tree, horse chestnut, laburnum, privet, and wisteria.

Porcupine Quills

Quills are used by porcupines to protect themselves from predators and from other kinds of danger that may occur. They are loosely attached and can be easily dislodged on contact. It is very fundamental to remove all quills carefully so as to prevent further damages and injuries to the cat. It is imperative to seek medical care for your cat immediately and have the quills removed while the cat has been subjected to general anesthesia.

Ensure no quills remain under the fur and skin of your cat as quills tend to break into small pieces which hide under the fur. A thorough examination is therefore required to solve this problem or situation.

Puncture Wounds

Bites from other cats, often leaving superficial skin wounds and creating a damp patch of matted hair, are the main causes of puncture wounds. Beneath the skin, discharge of puss may happen causing swelling and further infections throughout the body.

Bites to areas such as the abdomen can cause damage to organs as well as internal bleeding. Other examples of puncture wounds are if a sharp object penetrates the cat, for example, a nail from a fence, arrow or knife.

Abscesses tend to be very painful and cause distress to the cat as it builds up and prepares to burst and discharge pus. It is important to take the cat to a veterinary service for draining of the abscess and application of the suitable antibiotic.

If the abscess bursts on its own, clip the hair around the area and clean it with salt water. This is to kill germs and prevent any infection.

One should also apply pressure around the area to remove as much pus as possible and look for foreign objects such as seeds, splinters or grass.

In other situations abscesses can cause the cat to have fever and go off their food, usually the administration of antibiotics by a veterinary surgeon and possibly draining the abscess will assist a lot.

In cases where the cat has punctured its chest, cover the wound with a clean damp cloth and bandage the chest to seal the wound and seek immediate medical assistance.

Other important facts to note are as follows:

1. So as not to cause any fatal injuries, do not remove any objects that are still penetrating.
2. Air pellet injuries may be difficult to detect as they push the surrounding hair in the wound, on their entry.
3. If an arrow has penetrated into the skin of the cat, cut it 5cm from the cat's body, wrap tightly with a bandage around the point of entry so as to prevent further signs of injury and damage to the cat. Note that you should not remove such a penetrated object.

4. Monitor for signs of increased sensitivity to light and sound as this may be caused by tetanus, which is not common in cats but can thrive in cases of deep wounds.

Scratching

Allergic reactions and infestation with the Sarcoptes mite that causes scabies in humans can cause intense scratching leading to self-inflicted injury. Cats can have allergies to things they have ingested e.g. food medication, things they have had skin contact with e.g. stinging nettles washing powders or insects that have stung or bitten them e.g. wasp, bees or ants. Scratching can also be caused by infestations of fleas and mites and regular flea prevention with a product specifically designed for use in cats is recommended.

Look for signs of redness and Infection of the skin. If the skin seems normal, rinse the cat thoroughly with clean, warm water – do not add any shampoo or soap. Repeat this for two to three times, and then gently dry your cat. If scratching persists, or if the skin is in any way damaged, consult your veterinary officer.

Snake Bite

The severity of a snake bite varies with the species of snake, number of bites and amount of injected venom, especially in venomous snakes. Some certain type of snake venom attacks the nervous system, leading to seizures, weakness and coma. Viper bites make the area become black, and it is important to note that most bites are either on the face or the neck, as the cat tries to catch the snake.

Symptoms of a cat that is bitten by a snake are shock, unstable and uncoordinated cats. It is, therefore, important to relax your cat so as not to increase movement of the venom to other parts of the body and lastly, it is important to seek immediate veterinary advice.

Other measures to undertake include rinsing the wound, trying to remove as much of the venom as possible as you flush the wound with cool running water and apply a cold compress: this will assist in slowing blood circulation and prevent the poison spreading.

It will also help in reducing pain and swelling over the affected area. Keep the limb lower than the rest of the body if the cat has been bitten, as it more difficult for the venom to spread.

Spider Bites

Most spider bites are not poisonous. A non-venomous spider is characterized by seeing a small localized red mark at the area of the bite. Symptoms may include fever, shock, seizures, and paralysis in cases of venomous spider bites.

Examples of poisonous spiders include:

1. Black Widow, which is identified by a bright red circle on the abdomen. They are very dangerous and are the size of a large pea. They are also known for building webs in cool, dark places.
2. Brown Rescue Spider, which is identified by a violin shape on the chest. The bites from this spider causes death of tissue cells as they turn black and can lead to major infection if not treated immediately.

It is, therefore, important to, seek immediate medical advice if you realize that a spider has bitten your cat.

First steps to follow in cases of spider bites include: Keep your cat as quiet and relaxed as possible, any movement or excitement speeds up blood flow, therefore increasing movement of the venom to other body parts, seek immediate veterinary advice, rinse the wound, trying to remove as much of the venom as possible, flush the wound with cool running water, apply a cold compress: this slows down the spreading of the venom. It will also reduce pain and swelling. Lower the affected area: if you cat has been bitten on a limb, keep the limb lower than the rest of the body as this slows the spread of venom.

Swallowed Objects

During play time hours, kittens are more prone to ingest things that they shouldn't. These items are small enough to pass through the stomach and intestines, but some get stuck along the way. Once this happens, they cause blockages along the alimentary canal. Such obstructions cause retching or gagging depending on their location, and vomiting. Cats in such situations may experience loss of appetite and their feces may or may not continue to be passed depending on whether the obstruction is total or partial.

Of great concern are known as linear foreign bodies as these can cause the intestines to become concertinaed in a process called **enteroplication**.

Here, the cord cuts into the intestine and causes severe problems. If a large area of the intestine is involved the condition is fatal, and the cat is likely to die or need to be euthanized. It is, therefore, important to note that, in all cases of ingested foreign bodies, seek immediate veterinary help especially if your cat is showing sign of obstruction.

Swollen Paws

The most common causes of swollen paws are abscesses due to cat bites. Other cases of swollen paws can be checked by examining your cat, to remove any obvious bands or foreign bodies. Seek veterinary attention if the pus is frequent on swelling.

Urinary Problems

Due to the anatomy of their long thin urethras, male cats are prone to urinary tract blockages. Crystals and plugs of other materials can block the flow of urine from the bladder leading to discomfort, pain and rupture if not treated, and this can lead to shock and death.

Immediate medical services are required if the cat produces small amounts of urine, cries, visit the litter tray more often and show signs of strain.

A cat may experience a condition known as idiopathic cystitis, which is inflammation of the bladder either due to infection or presence of crystals. These cats are generally eating and otherwise normal but urinate more frequently and possibly inappropriately.

If you are able to obtain urine sample before you get to the vets this is of great assistance in trying to determine the underlying problem. Collect the sample in a clean container or use cotton wool to soak it up and put the sample inside a sealed plastic bag to retain moisture.

Vomiting

Licking, swallowing, and salivation are signs of nausea and impending vomiting. Cats often vomit to remove hairballs from their stomachs. Vomiting, however, can also indicate more serious conditions.

Seek immediate veterinary attention if the vomit is black, projectile, continuous or occurring in a kitten. If fever, restlessness, abdominal pain, bloody diarrhea or unsuccessful attempts to urinate are present, seek immediate veterinary help.

If the vomit is black, projectile, continuous or occurring in a kitten, seek immediate veterinary helo. If fever, restlessness, abdominal pain, bloody diarrhea or unsuccessful attempts to urinate are present, seek immediate veterinary help.

If the vomiting has occurred less than three times and is not accompanied by any other problems like diarrhea, withhold food for 12 hours and give small sips of water. Offer bland food like white fish or chicken – 1-2 teaspoonfuls every hour – if this is not vomited, offer a little more every 1-2hours.

If the vomiting has resolved, continue light feeding for 1-2 days then gradually re-introduce your cat's regular food. If a vomiting episode re-occurs, arrange to seek veterinary services.

OBSERVATION CHECKLIST FOR YOUR CAT

Notice if the cat is: alert, depressed, anxious, aggressive, increased and decrease of appetite as well as vomiting, increased and decreased thirst, hard, soft, liquid and bloody feces and varying urination patterns which are increased, decreased or inappropriate.

Also check for further signs such as: increased or decreased activity mobility, varying breathing behaviors, eye injuries, foul mouth and teeth and skin injuries as a result of penetration of foreign objects.

It is also essential to check for fleas and worms, the vaccination history of all animals that you tend to, or you keep in your house and lastly, increased temperatures as compared to when last checked. Therefore, it is required that one check for such conditions in cat regularly.

ITEMS NEEDED IN A FIRST AID KIT

Keep clean sealable plastic box or bag in a suitable container. Also pack cleaning materials such as cotton buds, wool, and sterile saline. In cases of injuries, equip yourself with, 7.5cm squared sterile non-stick gauze pads, 2.5cm and 5cm bandage for example Treat wrap, Conforming bandages such as Co-flex, 1cm adhesive tape, for example, a Microspore and a cotton wool role.

Further equipment is as follows: digital rectal thermometer, fine tip tweezers, nails clippers, Elizabeth collar, plastic gloves, a plastic syringe which is 5ml, eye dropper for eye injuries, traveling box and a towel and muzzle.

Medication

Medicine is also necessary when arranging your first aid kit. Examples of medicinal products to pack include: Over the counter eye drops for eye injuries which if left untreated can be very fatal, an ear cleaner for example Leo so as to clean the ears and remove bacteria, Liquid paraffin such as Katala, Kaolin mixture for example Kaogel, Water based sterile lubricant that is KY Jelly for applying on cuts and bruises, and feline shampoo e.g. Episoothe to induce vomiting.

List of information

It is also essential to carry with you a list of emergency contact numbers for your vet or out of hours service and a list of typical values of your cat's pulse, respiration rate, and temperature.

39063120R00036

Printed in Poland
by Amazon Fulfillment
Poland Sp. z o.o., Wrocław